Platinum Rules for Enjoying Life

ENDORSEMENTS FOR
Platinum Rules for Enjoying Life

Short, concise, and ripe for immediate application. These nourishing morsels are the perfect appetizer for living a life that is rich with purpose and fulfillment. The rules provided are not just theoretical musings but practical guidelines that can supercharge your life—today.

—**Dan Miller**, *New York Times* best-selling
author of *48 Days to the Work You Love*

Platinum Rules for Enjoying Life is the quintessential playbook to a lifetime of positive experiences. The book will lead you to be your BEST self, while having fun on the journey. It is a great guide and reminder that we create our own reality.

—**Julia Fox Garrison**, motivational speaker and
best-selling author of *Don't Leave Me This Way*

Platinum Rules for Enjoying Life brims with wisdom and insight into how we can be our best selves. These perfectly sized pieces of advice remind us to how to slow and savor, connect and appreciate.

—**Tova Mirvis**, best-selling author of
The Book of Separation

What a treasure trove these forty platinum rules are on how to bring more joy and fulfillment to each day! Each one uplifts our vision and enlivens confidence to act and do well, joyously, on what we wish of life and on what life asks of us. For my time-after-time go-to, *Platinum Rules for Enjoying Life* holds a special place in my home library.

—**Eleanor Brantley Schwartz**, Chancellor and Professor
Emerita, University of Missouri-Kansas City

This delightful book gives fascinating and encouraging ways to get more enjoyment and meaning in life. I love the first rule, "Laugh Often," as we need to give our lives a light touch. These platinum rules will help all of us be more flexible, positive, and content, valuing relationships, serving others, and finding our purpose. I thoroughly enjoyed this impactful book and hope you will too!

—**Rosemary Trible**, founder of Fear 2 Freedom, former First Lady of Christopher Newport University, and award-winning author of *Fear to Freedom*

This book was a great read for me. I've actually put a number of these practices in play already without knowing it. After reading *Platinum Rules for Enjoying Life*, I feel much more equipped to recognize what brings me joy now and learned some new ideas I can implement to grow a more balanced and fulfilling life. Thanks, Sylvia and Lisa!

—**Jeremy K. Franks**, Professional Golfers Association (PGA), owner of MyProGolfer24

Platinum Rules for Enjoying Life can be a catalyst for your happiness. You come home. It's been a pretty good day. You're in a thoughtful, contemplative mood. You begin to relax and perhaps take the measure of where you are in this journey called life. Here's what I love about what Sylvia and Lisa have done in creating *Platinum Rules for Enjoying Life*: This little book is a guide. The carefully thought-out sentiments come from a spiritual place. Just enjoy a few minutes with this book, and you'll discover that this is a catalyst for happiness. It nudges us to recognize the joy of where we have been and the mystery and intrigue of what is yet to come. And they subtly remind us, *don't waste a minute of it.*

—**Bud Ramey**, ghostwriter for *Forbes Books and* author of twelve nonfiction books

Life can be a joyful, frustrating, and complicated journey. But no matter how straightforward or complex, every journey requires a map, something that instructs on the best way to get where you want to be. In *Platinum Rules for Enjoying Life*, Sylvia Weinstein Craft and Lisa Spiller provide a step-by-step guide for navigating the emotional, spiritual, and intellectual challenges encountered in our humanly passage. Lisa and Sylvia have created an inspirational work that will become your dog-eared, worn-out reference guide. *Platinum Rules* is a must read for anyone seeking contentment, fulfillment, and true happiness.

—**David Perry**, best-selling author of
The Extern: A Jason Rodgers Novel

The authors of *Platinum Rules for Enjoying Life* draw from their years of personal and professional experiences in business, academe, marketing and community service to offer readers a comprehensive blueprint for bringing more passion, enjoyment, and satisfaction to their everyday lives. These rules serve as a foundation to provide practical advice and a vision to achieve a more complete life. While an easy read that offers time-tested tips such as "do unto others" and "tomorrow is another day," the book is very insightful reading that will challenge the mind, body, and soul. The gifted authors have prepared a remarkable book that can serve as a roadmap to a more fulfilling life. It should find a welcome home on one's coffee table or personal library.

—**Ronald J. Volpe**, President Emeritus, Hood College

No matter your age or current circumstances, *Platinum Rules for Enjoying Life* will surely enrich your life! Here are inspirational ideas you can implement immediately to improve your relationships, your health, your enjoyment of each and every day. Nuggets of wisdom are presented in an easy-to-access format to educate and inspire, no matter how busy your day. This is a book to keep close at hand for its many life-affirming benefits. Practical and encouraging . . . sure to brighten you and your loved ones' days.

—**Donna Baier Stein**, award-winning author
and publisher

Platinum Rules for Enjoying Life will change the way you live. It is a collection of simple yet powerful rules to help you live a happier, more fulfilling life. The book is written in a clear and concise style, and it is full of practical advice that you can start using right away. One of the things that I love about this book is the authors have spent their life studying and practicing the principles shared in the book. As a result, they are able to offer real-world advice to use to make a difference in your life. If you are looking for a book to help you to live a happier, more fulfilling life, I highly recommend this book. It will change the way you think about life and give you the tools you need to make a difference.

—**Douglas Fry**, executive director at
Association of Community Publishers

Platinum Rules for Enjoying Life is a beautiful reminder that it is not complicated to live a healthy life full of gratitude, patience, deep friendships and more. This book shows us how we can accomplish a full and balanced life simply by changing how we think and act. A wonderful read!

—**Amy Hart**, owner and president of Hauser's Jewelers

Henry Wadsworth Longfellow once said "Simplicity in character, in manners, in style—in all things the supreme excellence is simplicity." Sylvia and Lisa have written a book that's simplicity in style and supreme in excellence. If you want to learn the rules to living a life of excellence, pick up, read, and apply the *Platinum Rules for Enjoying Life*.

—**Charles M. Taylor**, CEO/lead coach
at Charles and Shakira Unlimited

This is truly a book for all seasons of our lives—and for people of all ages. Read it through the first time to enjoy the engaging writing. You will happily find many positive and helpful "rules." Then go back, time and time again, to individual sections for inspiration and concrete advice. It will become your manual and trusted source for directions and encouragement. Congratulations to authors Craft and Spiller for giving us a companion that reminds us how fulfilling life can be.

—**Elizabeth Young**, professor and author of six books,
including *Do You See Him Now?* and *Finding J. Hubbard*

Everyone wants to live the "good life," but too often the focus turns to chasing external rewards beyond our control. In *Platinum Rules for Enjoying Life*, Sylvia Weinstein Craft and Lisa Spiller nudge readers toward inward thought practices that build a rich life from the inside out. This snappy read offers perspectives on self-improvement, time management, healthy living, and relishing the rhythms of the calendar year with takeaway maxims that can improve life in tangible, present-tense ways. Think of this little book as a field guide for navigating the path toward the fulfillment we all crave.

—**Cynthia Vacca Davis**, author of *Intersexion:
Story of Faith, Identity, and Authenticity*

Platinum Rules for Enjoying Life shares timeless wisdom presented in bite-sized morsels. It reminds me of the enduring principles our grandparents shared with us, passed down through the generations but often forgotten in today's hustle and bustle. Each concept is easy to read and quick to consume but will leave you pondering ways to improve and enjoy life more. It will inspire you to reflect on lessons of the past that can still be applied to today's opportunities. Ultimately, *Platinum Rules for Enjoying Life* encourages you to live each day with joy and significance.

—**Charles George**, entrepreneur, publisher, and direct marketer at Publish to Thrive

Simple yet profoundly impactful self-help book for those who want to improve the quality of their life's journey. What is a reminder for some will be new insights for another. No matter what age reader, this book is an encouraging resource that is much needed in current times.

—**Michele Savaunah Zirkle**, author, inspirational speaker, life coach, spiritual teacher

Ingenious and resourceful! This book encapsulates such profound practical points for guiding us to live a more fulfilling, fun, meaningful life, yet we overlook and/or do not apply them. It reminded me of the importance of a simple human touch, how to have a quick comeback at an embarrassing memory lapse and then laugh at yourself, that prayer is food for the soul, how giving is itself enriching, and many more! Thanks to the authors, two well-respected women, Sylvia Weinstein Craft and Lisa D. Spiller, for sharing your insightful rules that help us live our best life!

—**Lois B. Boyle**, executive director at Access Virginia

Sylvia Weinstein Craft and Lisa Spiller have crafted a delightful road map for living your best life. Readers will also get some gentle reminders that we only get one life to get it right. *Platinum Rules for Enjoying Life* is chock-full of bite-sized examples and tips that you'll want to keep handy so you can leaf through it anytime you're in need of inspiration or advice.

—**Beverly McLean**, CTC, Covington
International Travel

Platinum Rules for Enjoying Life certainly outlines a very easy way for self-care. It's a great road map for self-exploration to a wonderful conclusion. I would definitely recommend reading this inspirational book often.

—**Bob Kessler**, former executive director at United
Jewish Community of the Virginia Peninsula

Platinum Rules for Enjoying Life puts in perspective the overlooked, simple joys that life can offer. It reminds people that the golden rule is the basis of a successful, happy, loving, peaceful life for themselves and everyone around them. It is a book you can pick up and reread just to keep yourself aware and grounded, remembering to be thankful for every day and with a little awareness to live your best God-given life! THANK YOU!

—**Ann Sears**, entrepreneur and part-owner
of Style by Design

Platinum Rules for Enjoying Life is a heartfelt, down-to-earth read that is filled with takeaways to live by. Authors Craft and Spiller have put the big picture in perspective with their tried-and-true *carpe diem* advice. Reading this book is habit-forming. Keep it within reach.

—**Susan Zimmerman**, freelance travel and history writer

I found *Platinum Rules for Enjoying Life* very refreshing and uplifting—a great reminder of years past and today's world—things I once did and no longer do. Your book brought it all back in place. Life can be so complicated these days as changes take place through the years. It was like an awakening in my life! I see great book gifts ahead for family and friends.

—**Nancy B. Alligood**, CTC, Warwick Travel Service

This enlightening book matches well with my basic philosophy of how I've lived each of my ninety-nine years of life! The forty rules align with my "ACE Factor," which stands for attitude, conviction, and enthusiasm. I can connect with every word in *Platinum Rules for Enjoying Life*.

—**Dorothy "Dot" Knopf**, Newport News, Virginia

Platinum Rules
for
Enjoying Life

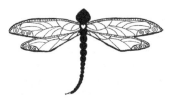

Sylvia Weinstein Craft
Lisa D. Spiller

NEW YORK

LONDON • NASHVILLE • MELBOURNE • VANCOUVER

Platinum Rules *for* Enjoying Life

Published in New York, New York, by Morgan James Publishing. Morgan James is a trademark of Morgan James, LLC. www.MorganJamesPublishing.com

Proudly distributed by Publishers Group West®

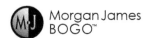

Morgan James BOGO™

A **FREE** ebook edition is available for you or a friend with the purchase of this print book.

CLEARLY SIGN YOUR NAME ABOVE

Instructions to claim your free ebook edition:
1. Visit MorganJamesBOGO.com
2. Sign your name CLEARLY in the space above
3. Complete the form and submit a photo of this entire page
4. You or your friend can download the ebook to your preferred device

ISBN 9781636982144 paperback
ISBN 9781636982151 ebook
Library of Congress Control Number: 2023937544

Cover and Interior Design by:
Chris Treccani
www.3dogcreative.net

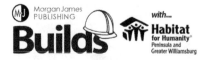

Morgan James PUBLISHING Builds

with... **Habitat for Humanity®** Peninsula and Greater Williamsburg

Morgan James is a proud partner of Habitat for Humanity Peninsula and Greater Williamsburg. Partners in building since 2006.

Get involved today! Visit: www.morgan-james-publishing.com/giving-back

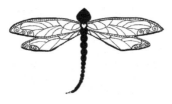

From:

Contents

Acknowledgments

As authors, we are personally responsible for the content in this book; however, we happily acknowledge the valuable input and assistance from several individuals. While writing this book, we were flanked by some very thoughtful and giving people.

Our warmest gratitude to Lisa's sister, Cathy DiSalvo, who competently edited the content of each of the 40 Rules and offered so many valuable suggestions and insight. She is surely earning her wings for heaven!

We are truly thankful to Sylvia's daughter, Lorri Hanna, for designing the unique and beautiful dragonfly image used throughout our book.

Grateful appreciation to Philip Burcher, wordsmith and writer, who initially crafted and created many of the thoughts and words that became our Rules.

Special thanks to fitness guru Brian Cole, owner of Personal Training Associates, for helping us develop our Rules for Healthy Living.

We are most grateful to Cathy Welch, photographer extraordinaire, for working with us on our author photograph.

Sincere thanks to our editor, Claudia Volkman of Creative Editorial Solutions, for her efficient and competent professional assistance.

We extend genuine gratitude for the valuable insight, wonderful support, and helpful assistance provided by David Hancock, founder of Morgan James Publishing, and his highly skilled team, including Naomi Chellis, Addy Normann, Jim Howard, and Bethany Marshall.

Lastly, we are forever grateful for the love and support we have received from our family members and friends while working on this book.

Introduction

More rules? Seriously? No way! Why read a book about rules when you may feel that there are already too many rules governing your life? Nobody needs more rules, right? And yet, everyone needs the 40 Rules contained in this little book. *Platinum Rules for Enjoying Life* will help you to stay on track to living a fulfilling and rewarding life. These Rules are designed to remind us to live each day to the fullest and to the best of our ability as we are not guaranteed a tomorrow.

In case you're wondering how this book came to be, here's our unique story. Most of the content contained in this book was extracted from decades of previously published columns appearing in *Oyster Pointer,* an independently published monthly newspaper. Though never called rules, pieces of advice were embedded into columns for a wide array of topics. Sylvia's dear friend Lisa remarked several times how much she enjoyed reading these columns and suggested that the content would make an inspirational book on living life to the fullest. The combination of the advice contained in the published columns and Lisa's vision and organization enabled the authors to create the content that appears in this little book!

While our book contains forty helpful reminders and bits of advice—many of which you've likely heard through the years—it's not an all-inclusive collection. We're sure that you've had unique experiences and valuable lessons learned regarding "enjoying life" that you can pass along.

We encourage you to list your favorite rules for life in the notes section at the back of the book.

Perhaps most advice books like this one have been lived before they were written. This is true for most, if not all, of the forty Platinum Rules that we suggest. While we can't claim that we've applied these rules perfectly in every situation, we certainly strive to do so, and feel happier when we do! And now you can too!

May our forty Platinum Rules enhance the joy and contentment you receive by living each day to the fullest and creating a life of significance!

Part One:

Rules for Self-Improvement

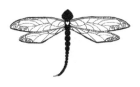

Rule 1:

Laugh Often

We all love a big happy smile! That's when one's face is the most radiant. A simple smile has the power to change someone's whole day. Additionally, a smile is a prelude to laughter. From a light snicker to an earsplitting roar, there's not much that is more therapeutic than a good laugh, and it's totally free!

The *Britannica Dictionary* defines *laughter* as "the action or sound of laughing, which is an expression of emotion, usually joy, mirth, or scorn." When you react to stimuli in the form of laughter, it is an outward sign of an engaging sense of humor.

Moreover, many experts in human behavior believe that laughter relaxes the entire body, and a good laugh relieves physical tension and alleviates stress. Some experts also suggest that laughter protects the heart by improving the function of blood vessels and increasing blood flow, both helpful in preventing cardiovascular problems such as heart attacks.

When you laugh, doesn't it make you feel good all over? Laughter can be contagious, binding people from all walks of life together in a common circle of joy.

Each morning, be determined to find humor throughout the day and cheer up those around you. Enjoy watching their faces brighten up!

Finally, laugh out loud. Laugh at anything that strikes you as funny and notice how much better you feel. Remember that laughter can change the world, one person at a time.

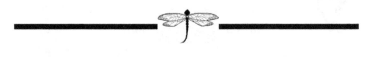

Takeaway:

LOL = Laugh Out Loud!

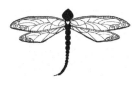

Rule 2:

Express Gratitude

Thank you: These two words carry so much power. In all aspects of life, this simple statement acknowledges gratitude for both small and large gifts, whether tangible or intangible. Thank you for being my friend, for listening and understanding. Thank you for making dinner, for the lovely flowers. The list is endless!

Do you find it fascinating that even those who are not multilingual invariably know this expression of appreciation in foreign tongues? Most everyone knows *merci, gracias, danke,* and other variations of this universal phrase. This means that almost everyone around the globe can use this simple form of speech to express appreciation for the many kindnesses in life.

Our Golden Rule (Treat others as you would wish to be treated) always promotes gratitude, and it is an ideal motto to live by. It encourages us to care for and respect all people, and it sets the stage for both giving and receiving simple favors and moral support.

Beyond the sending of a thank-you note, e-mail, or text message, appreciation can be expressed with personal gifts or donations in memory or in honor of someone's kindness.

Can you imagine a world in which we did not help one another? It would signal the end of the best characteristic of humanity. We need to receive kindness as much as we need to give it. It's in our very nature. Unfortunately, too often in the busyness of our lives, we postpone or fail to express our appreciation for the kindness of others.

So, let's make expressing gratitude a priority, and show it more often.

Takeaway:

Use those two powerful little words!

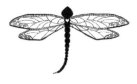

Rule 3:

Overcome Awkward Moments

L ife is full of surprises! One minute you're basking on a sandy shore, safe, sound, and blissful, and the next minute, you're tossing around like a ship on a stormy sea. Typically, these unexpected and difficult moments require more grace and social skills than we can muster instantaneously.

Indeed, life often places us in unpredictable situations. For example, you are shopping with a lifelong friend when you hear your name being called from across the shop by a business associate. You make the usual hi-how-are-you's, and when you go to introduce your friend, life doles out a surprise. "I'd like you to meet my dear friend, err . . ." Your mind goes completely blank—a very embarrassing blank! Fortunately, she comes to your rescue and introduces herself, but you remain embarrassed, wondering what just happened.

Life really keeps us on our toes. You may be able to relate to the above scenario with an "err" moment of your own. Hopefully, it was not of great consequence and the outcome was laughter and understanding. Whether our brains get distracted or overloaded, it's easy to experience momentary memory lapses.

The lesson we learn from these awkward moments is that a sense of humor comes to our rescue. When that "err" moment strikes, be honest, sincere, and ready with a joke. Being able to laugh at ourselves helps overcome our embarrassment, allowing us to get through the situation with poise and sincerity.

Ah, life! How we meet its smaller challenges makes us who we are and enables us to respond well when bigger challenges come our way.

Takeaway:

Roll with the punches!

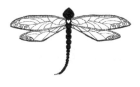

Rule 4:

Practice Patience

Aren't we always complaining about how busy we are? In the electronic age, computers have been instrumental in making our expectations of productivity so high. Now, even computers are too slow for many people.

Today, we can accomplish instantly what would have taken hours years ago. So, what does this mean to our daily lives? In a word, momentum. We've become accustomed to working fast, moving fast, thinking fast. Even when our bodies are still, our minds can still be racing.

Momentum is everywhere! Watch someone push an elevator button repeatedly, as if it will make the doors open sooner. Or watch the line-jumper in the market, who goes from one line to another in hopes of a shorter wait, only to be stopped by someone needing a price check. And then, there's the ATM line, with people shifting from one foot to another because thirty seconds is too long to wait for cash!

Surely, you've experienced the irritated driver who curses the traffic signal or blasts the horn the second the light changes. Or the interstate driver who weaves from lane to lane until he gets ahead of the pack. And there's always someone complaining to a waiter when service feels too slow.

Patience, we know, is a virtue, but it's a practiced virtue. Are we forgetting to practice?

Recognize opportunities to practice patience instead of focusing on the annoyance you may feel. Slow down. Relax. Go with the flow. Chill out. You may soon discover that you can feel contentment, even in the face of annoying situations.

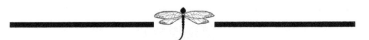

Takeaway:

Relax and enjoy a tranquil ride!

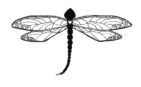

Rule 5:

Listen to Your Inner Voice

J ust imagine, you are gliding through the supermarket aisles where so many temptations call out to you from the displays, shelves, refrigerators, and freezers. Let's face it, indulging ourselves can lead to strong momentary pleasure. This is true regardless of whether our desire is for food, drink, or activities we most enjoy.

Every day there are temptations in life that plague us. If we consistently indulged them fully, we'd become quite imbalanced. Luckily, we have a little voice within us, perhaps, our inner conscience that cautions us to temper our response to cravings and desires.

Your inner voice encourages you to go for a walk to keep healthy and keeps you from making too many trips to the cookie jar. Your little voice helps you to make smart choices and can keep you out of all sorts of trouble. It plays a significant part in your enjoyment of life.

Your inner voice may seem to deprive you of life's indulgences and exquisite momentary pleasures. Do you ever talk back to your little voice? Perhaps you argue with it and say, "These extra treats won't make a significant difference!" But that little voice knows your habits and tendencies and guides you toward what's best in the grand scheme of your life.

To more fully enjoy life, you need to come to good terms with your little voice. Learn to appreciate it and heed its advice. Become friends with it and you may realize that it supports you enjoying all your favorite things in moderation throughout your life.

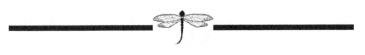

Takeaway:

Trust your conscience!

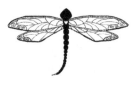

Rule 6:

Avoid Perfectionism

"It looks just great, except . . ." Do you begin sentences in this manner? Are you often unsatisfied with your performance? If so, don't look now, but you could be suffering from perfectionism!

Many of us want to be the very best in all that we do. Unfortunately, if you spend more time striving for perfection rather than achieving your goals, you may be driving yourself and your family and friends "perfectly" crazy while you miss out on some of the joy in life.

Some ways to identify that you're teetering on the brink of perfectionism are being told you're "nitpicky," obsessing over small, pointless details, feeling unable to delegate tasks to others or being disappointed when you can't finish your "to-do" lists.

Perfectionism is insidious and the desire for complete control can spread into all areas of your life. To avoid this, decide at the start of an activity what an acceptable outcome looks like, then spend the shortest amount of time to achieve it.

Remember that we all make mistakes; then learn to trust yourself and others. Accept that solid effort and very good results may be enough. Few activities warrant the time and energy needed to strive for perfection.

Above all, put some perspective on the true importance of things and "lighten up!" Chances are you'll soon find yourself content and still successful.

Takeaway:

Find contentment in good results!

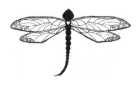

Rule 7:

Appreciate Your Age

Have you ever noticed that young people want to be older? What young person doesn't long for the day when he or she can get a driver's license, or be of legal drinking age? For all those yearning for adulthood, we just want to put our arms around them and say, "Be your age. Enjoy youth, innocence, and the lack of adult responsibilities."

Maybe you're still in your twenties and feel you have everything ahead of you. And yet, where has your childhood gone? Pause for a moment and reminisce about what you loved most during your youth. Consider how to build on your successes as well as learn and grow from your mistakes.

Many of us remember a bit of trauma in turning thirty, forty, fifty, or sixty. We learn, albeit slowly, to accept our ages and to appreciate the honor (yes, honor!) of being blessed with longevity. We recognize that advancing age brings us a broader perspective on things and a certain wisdom we didn't have in our youth.

Let's not bother to delve into all the clichés that have become a part of our daily conversation. Yes, age is just a number, and technically, a birthday is just another day.

And, to those adults who dread birthdays, realize that every stage of life brings new experiences to enjoy. Learn to be thankful for the gift of life and the blessings granted throughout the entire adventure.

At each stage, reflect on your new strengths, enhanced abilities, and amazing revelations about yourself. Continue to grow by seeking new experiences along the way.

Takeaway:

Celebrate each birthday!

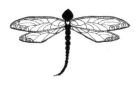

Rule 8:

Seize Success

Learning to ride a bicycle? Earning your first A+ or receiving praise for an excellent presentation? Do you remember the first time you experienced that marvelous feeling known as success?

At that time, you caught the trapeze bar and glided through the tent-topped air of recognition and accomplishment for a performance that was better than anyone else had done, perhaps even better than you dreamed of. It's what most of us strive for.

Success around the workplace is often considered as financial or professional advancements, and more responsibility. You've likely heard the motivational gurus tout "go the extra mile, work the extra hour, out-perform your peers." But have you considered your own definition of success?

A feeling of success is important throughout your life. Success can be your first homemade apple pie, teaching your two-year-old the alphabet, or getting your driver's license. Success can result from learning new skills, developing our innate abilities, serving our families, and contributing to our communities.

In all areas of our lives, success fuels our drive, ambition, and get-up-and-go. It's the carrot that keeps us striving to do more. One of the best ways to recognize our success is to break large projects or goals into subtasks and celebrate our success as each step is completed.

From the boardroom to the kitchen, from the classroom to the garage, success is within our reach when we work for it. So, when you achieve your goals, savor the moment and revel in the glory of your hard-earned success!

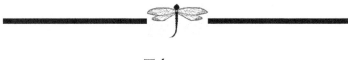

Takeaway:

You can do it!

Part Two:

Rules for Spending Time

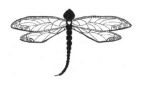

Rule 1:

Manage Time

In case you haven't noticed, life these days is moving entirely too fast. Regardless of our age, this frantic, fast-paced lifestyle has touched everyone. We rarely give ourselves a break.

We are overworked, overbooked, and overdue for a few minutes of some peace and quiet or for hours of serenity. We're missing that euphoria of nothingness when the mind and the body meet as one and we can actually take a break and breathe deeply. We simply need to slow down in order to savor life, like we would a fine wine.

It sure is tempting to try to get as much as possible done. We make a list and allot time for each task on it. Then we scurry around as if being timed on a stopwatch. We fail to recognize that what we don't complete will be waiting for us tomorrow.

So, take a refreshing walk in the woods. Read a good book or browse through some magazines. Leisurely write letters. Take that long-overdue nap or just rest quietly for a while. You'll find that once you're properly rested, you'll actually get more done in the long run.

Life is to be enjoyed. Take time to reflect on how much you love your friends and family. Look around and marvel at a rainbow or a snowflake. Feel the sun's warmth or a cool gentle breeze. *Ahhhhh . . .*

The race won't take its toll on you if you're not running in it, so enjoy a stroll instead. You'll probably live longer and feel more at peace with yourself and the world around you.

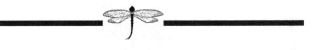

Takeaway:

Slow down and relax!

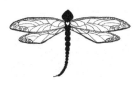

Rule 2:

Stay Focused

While washing dishes, you remember that you need to pay a bill. You go into your home office and notice a sticky note reminding you to place an online order. You sit down at your computer and see two emails awaiting your response. Isn't it easy to get sidetracked? Before you know it, your bill has not been paid, the dishwater is cold, and you wonder where the afternoon has gone.

Has multitasking ruined our lives? Are you no longer able to stick with one task at a time, or do you often feel like a bouncing ball taking on everything in your path, but not accomplishing what you intended to do?

Have you ever walked into a room to get something, forgotten what it was, but are sure you'll recognize the item when you see it?

The age of technology has completely revolutionized the way we do things. With information and time-saving hacks so readily available, we overestimate how much we can complete in a given amount of time. We may make to-do lists, prioritize our actions, and arrange our schedules in a logical order and then plunge into getting things done. But we often get sidetracked! It happens to all of us!

Sometimes it can take enormous effort to keep your mind focused on what is directly in front of you at the moment. Try to narrow your focus and complete one task at a time. And, believe it or not, you'll still get things done—one task at a time. Yes, you are still multitasking, but in a more directed way.

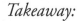

Takeaway:

Prioritize and focus on one task at a time!

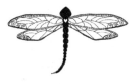

Rule 3:

Respect Routines, but Stay Flexible

Errrrnnn . . . errrnnn . . . there goes the alarm! Both feet on the floor for another day. You brush your teeth; jump into workout clothes; check your phone for weather, messages, and emails; then out the door for some early exercise. Return home, shower, get dressed, check traffic, and drive to work.

Most of us have set routines that we follow, at least on weekdays. These activities are done in the proper sequence and become automatic habits that serve us well on most days. They provide a sense of order and keep us moving toward meeting our goals.

But could these routines actually become a detriment to your enjoyment of life? Routines can rob you of your sense of adventure when you shop at the same stores, watch the same TV programs, eat the same foods, and stay safely in your comfort zone at all times.

What's the alternative? Stray from your comfort zone periodically and allow each day to be unique. Between sunrise and sunset, experience something new each day. You may even emerge with a new favorite food, store, show, or activity. Then, modify your routine going forward to include new favorites and build confidence in your flexibility.

Let's face it—life can be challenging sometimes. There are times when life catches us off guard and our well-tested routine fails to accommodate the unexpected. But if we've been practicing flexibility in our daily lives, we will be able to pivot readily when situations throw us a curveball.

So, refine your routine periodically and enjoy the variety of options available to you each day.

Takeaway:

Variety is the spice of life!

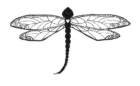

Rule 4:

Simplify Your Life

Have you ever wondered how "to do" lists came to be? Back in the days before Post-it Notes were invented, many of us saw our mother create simple grocery lists on a lined notepad and check off each item as she added it to her cart. Taken to the next step, she labeled another page "Get it done today." This sheet included tasks such as wash dishes, call plumber, make lunches, and schedule lunch with Linda.

Post-it Notes expanded our lists and were stuck on kitchen cabinets, bathroom mirrors, the front door, and even the steering wheel of our cars. Soon this blizzard of Post-its coalesced into notes on our cell phones. How convenient to be able to copy and paste additional chores from one day to the next!

Today, our list for one day may contain things such as workout at the fitness center, have nails done, pick up dry cleaning, get gas for car, make bank deposit, write thank-you notes, bake cookies, and attend a neighborhood association meeting. Unfortunately, we fail to notice that the items on today's list take much longer than fulfilling a simple grocery list did. Yet we expect ourselves to complete the whole list in a day.

Do you ever dream of deleting your to-do list or calendar? While we can't do that, we can combine multiple trips into one, ask family members to do one task each, limit our purchases to have fewer things to care for, prioritize activities, and set realistic expectations for ourselves. We can vow not to overbook ourselves and to schedule in a few breaks for reflecting, dreaming, and relaxing.

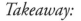

Takeaway:

Lighten today's load . . . tomorrow's another day!

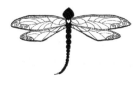

Rule 5:

Relish Reading

A re you an avid reader? Do you enjoy curling up with a book or an iPad and losing yourself in the power and color of words? Have you ever transported your spirit to a farm in Africa, a white-sand beach in Florida, or a swanky New York nightclub?

What a wonderful break from the routine of our days! A good book keeps our imaginations alive and take us away from grocery lists, dental appointments, work pressures, and our daily tasks.

As you know, books can go anywhere with us. Books require no wires and plugs, no fuel, no handles, no clips, no cumbersome cases. They fly well, relax well on beaches, and flourish in waiting rooms and cafes. The same can be true for online and audiobooks!

And what a prism of personalities books offer! Mysteries that keep us up late, romances that fill us with tears, biographies that bring people alive, advice and self-help books that spark ideas and fresh perspectives, and the list goes on.

Books offer a world swirling with adventures beyond our more ordinary lives. Books convey plots that keep us guessing, word power that expands our vocabulary, fields of new ideas to explore and inspire us, and most of all, marvelous entertainment.

So, find your happy place and let your mind go for a magical ride in a good book. Reading is a simple joy that has endless pleasures. Rest assured that your to-do list will still be waiting for you when you emerge from your escape to that amazing Hawaiian Island. You may find that you have renewed energy for your day-to-day demands once you return!

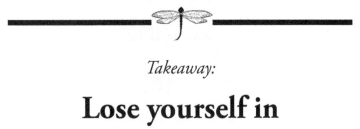

Takeaway:

Lose yourself in a good book!

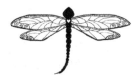

Rule 6:

Pray and Reflect

Most of us just pray for God to help us or to bless us. And unfortunately, because of our busy lives, prayer is often an afterthought. But what is prayer and why is it important?

Praying is the most intimate form of communication that directly connects us to God on a personal level. Praying reminds us that we are not alone, that God is always at our side.

Prayer can be done by groups as well as individuals. When we pray, we welcome God into our lives and become closer to Him. In prayer, we put our trust in God and ask Him to intervene in our lives or the lives of others.

Praying is simple—just speak to Him with a genuine heart. This can be done anywhere, anytime! You may pray that God's wisdom helps you decide how to respond to a request, pray just to thank Him, or pray for peace when you feel overwhelmed.

In prayer, we can recognize God's miracles and rely on His infinite power. We can feel an inner peace despite things going on around us! And even when we're not sure what to pray for, God knows what we need, and He always answers our prayers. Sometimes His answer in any given moment may not be what we wished for, but we can rest assured that He sees a much bigger picture and knows what is truly best for each of us.

So, regardless of how you are feeling, spend time praying and reflecting to anchor yourself in the peace of God's love for you.

Takeaway:

Pray and reflect to deepen your relationship with God.

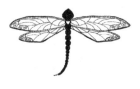

Rule 7:

Refresh Yourself

If you're looking at pie charts but seeing pyramids along the Nile or if you're undeniably exhausted at the end of the day, you may be ready for a vacation. If your morning shower has you dreaming of a Hawaiian waterfall, you're absolutely ready.

Have you ever considered a vacation as running out on your fellow workers or neglecting your daily duties? Or perhaps you've wondered how you could relax on a beach with a report due and that monthly meeting on your calendar. Just dispel those thoughts! Vacations are essential to your well-being because they whisk away the daily routine and allow you to more fully relax.

Rest assured, life will go on and work will get done while you're sipping sangrias in Mexico, surfing in Costa Rica, golfing in South Carolina, lounging on a beach, climbing an Alp, learning the hula, getting a new you at a spa, or just sitting under an umbrella in your backyard. Today you can take a trip around the world in a week. While that might not be the most relaxing vacation, it's surely filled with excitement!

Of course, when you say, "I'm never going back," it's time to do just that. Get back to work. Because you are refreshed and energized, you may have a new outlook on life—and work.

So, let yourself go! Cure the doldrums with new people, places, and activities. The world out there is really exciting and full of surprises. Treat yourself! Indulge! There's nothing like a vacation to give you new perspectives on how to enjoy life.

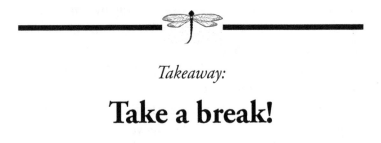

Takeaway:

Take a break!

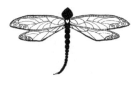

Rule 8:

Cherish Life

The older we get, the more joyful experiences we have to look back on. We may also find that certain memories are too important to ever forget.

Keeping a journal or diary is one good way to preserve and organize your memories. Keeping morsels of memorabilia, such as your children's kindergarten artwork, notes from friends, and photographs make great "memory joggers." Revisiting them transports you to another time or place in a process called daydreaming. Daydreams take your mind off daily duties and responsibilities and channel you into your own private world of nostalgia, dreams, and aspirations.

The simplest things, such as an aroma or an image, can elicit a memory of long ago, bringing it alive again. Daydreams can be warm, safe, and soothing to the soul or reminders of what we've learned from past mistakes. Daydreaming keeps us in touch with who we are and what has shaped our lives.

Have you filled albums, hard drives, or a cloud with old photos and memorabilia? If so, browse through them and allow the surge of nostalgia to sweep over you. Relive the times when you, your friends, and your loved ones were close together and supporting one another through both the best and worst of times.

And what could be more nourishing to the soul than getting together with an old friend and daydreaming together? That's when the laughter rises to a crescendo! You remain important to each other, bonded for life by those old, sweet memories.

We all have beautiful memories from many moments in our lives. Take the time to cherish and keep them alive by sharing them with friends and loved ones.

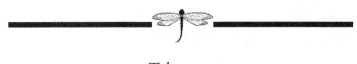

Takeaway:

Relive life's precious moments!

Part Three:

Rules for Enhancing Relationships

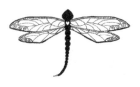

Rule 1:

Learn to Trust

Have you ever stopped to consider how many relationships you've made through the course of your life? Think about it. You have relationships with your God, family members, and friends, but you also have relationships with your doctor, dentist, banker, hairstylist, plumber, grocer, etc.

Whether it's shaped like a heart, a contract, or a ball and chain, a human relationship is simply a connection between people. You form relationships with all those people with whom you interact on a regular basis. You get to know them and then decide about trusting. When both people offer their full attention, affection, genuine concern, and ability to maintain confidences with each other, an honorable relationship is formed. Having good relationships with the people you interact on a regular basis contributes to your sense of well-being, peacefulness, success, happiness, and enjoyment of life.

Your relationships, built on trust, are what makes life worth living. Take time to nourish these relationships, step back and reshape them when needed, and even put them to the test on occasion. You will see that relationships with a solid foundation will remain unshakable.

So, reflect on the trusted people in your life and the relationships that give it depth and meaning. Connect often with them to show that you care and to let them know how you feel about them. Show kindness and respect in all of your relationships so that others view you as their trusted friend and confidante.

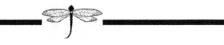

Takeaway:

Remain trustworthy!

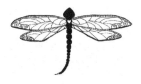

Rule 2:

Support Your Friends

Second only to the *Golden Rule*, "Do unto others as you would have them do unto you," is the maxim "A friend in need is a friend indeed." Yet too often we hear that when people are in trouble or have tragedies in their lives, friends may seem to be scarce; hence the term *fair-weather friends*.

Most of us experience friendship on a variety of different levels. We may have acquaintances who we really like, casual friends we get together with every few weeks or months, and best friends who enrich our lives on a daily basis. To be a true friend to someone is to stand by them, whatever crisis may burden them, through thick and thin, in sickness and in health. And if that sounds familiar, it should. The promises of friendship are strikingly similar to wedding vows (without the twenty-four hour/day commitment!) True friends give our lives meaning and substance and can help us navigate through life's difficulties.

Perhaps right now a friend of yours is struggling due to illness or some other challenge. Don't worry if you don't know what to do or say; your friend may not know either.

Reach out with a message that just says, "I'm here when you need me" or "What can I do to help you?" A simple expression of affection and support is better than a literary masterpiece.

Reflect on the value of the friendship and offer encouraging words and acts of kindness when needed. Remember that there is joy in giving and allow others to assist you in your time of need as well!

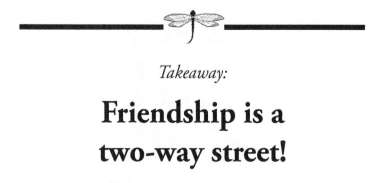

Takeaway:

Friendship is a two-way street!

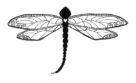

Rule 3:

Reconnect with Friends

In the adventure of life, there are many choices. What route is the fastest? Turn left or right at the fork in the road? Though we enjoy the scenery along our chosen path, we may be surprised to find that the strength of our relationships with people met along the way determines our quality of life.

Yes, we all make friends outside of our family. They are just as important because we actively choose them instead of "inheriting" them. We select our friends based on mutual respect and emotional connection. They are the people we value to share our lives. We understand and accept one another's strengths and weaknesses, and we can laugh and cry, learn and grow together.

Do you have friends from old neighborhoods, high school, college, or former workplaces? Do you still communicate with them? If you have you lost contact with someone special, resolve to connect again! Get out your old address book, click through your electronic contact list, or search Facebook for those long-lost friends.

It's so rewarding to spend time writing notes, sending e-mails or text messages, connecting on a social media platform, or perhaps calling people who are etched fondly in our memories. Enjoy reconnecting and reminiscing about special times you had together. Don't be surprised if the conversation leads you to connecting with more old friends. Staying in touch with friends from the past is likely to enrich you and enhance your appreciation of your personal development throughout life's journey.

So, reach out and reconnect with the people who've mattered the most and significantly impacted your life.

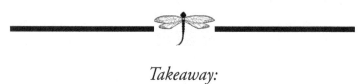

Takeaway:

Look them up!

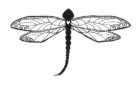

Rule 4:

Write and Save Notes

There's power in the written word. A congratulatory note, a thank-you, a holiday sentiment, an expression of sympathy—notes convey our thoughts with just the right words. A handwritten note is a personal gesture that warms the soul of both the sender and the recipient.

Note writing was ingrained in many of us from our childhood days when we would dutifully write notes to friends and relatives after receiving birthday or holiday gifts. And many of us still take pleasure in both writing and receiving them as these notes often contain our deepest feelings about the recipient, things we may struggle to say in casual, daily encounters.

Have you saved any notes that you have received? Have there been warm notes of appreciation, thoughtful pearls of wisdom, or meaningful messages that you just cannot crumple and toss? These notes are part of your history! They bring back memories of friends and family, some perhaps no longer with us on earth. Just seeing the handwriting of people who've gone before you can draw them closer to you in spirit. Reading old notes can remind you of happy times and rekindle such warm and loving feelings that you feel special all over again! Personal notes can be thought of as a warm and fuzzy indulgence. They are emotionally nourishing and one of the simple pleasures of life.

One of these days, your loved ones will review your collection of notes and may gain more insight than they had before. Notes sent to others, as well as those you've saved, are a lasting reminder of the love you experienced throughout your life.

Takeaway:

Write your heart out!

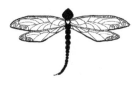

Rule 5:

Communicate Effectively

E ffective communication is the key to successful relationships! Perhaps a cliché, but a valid one.

Communication is the exchange of thoughts, information, ideas, and messages between people or groups. But it's not effective communication unless the sender's intent is properly understood by the receiver. Communication may be verbal, nonverbal (through expression and behavior), or written (by hand or electronically.)

In conversation, most of us focus so narrowly on selecting the "right" words that we tend to ignore the even more important aspects of our body language and tone of voice. Be sure your tone, body language, and message are in sync in order to convey precisely what you want to communicate.

To communicate effectively, try to adopt the seven C's of communication. Ensure that your message is clear (states exactly what is intended), concise (states thoughts and ideas as briefly as possible), concrete (provides facts to support your thoughts), correct (accurate both factually and grammatically), coherent (details logically centers around your main point), complete (provides all relevant information you want to convey), and courteous (shows honesty, respect, and friendliness). Communicating effectively will likely strengthen your relationships with others by ensuring that your messages are well received and properly understood. After an important discussion, always ask the recipient what message he or she took away from the conversation. If that understanding differs from your intention, discuss the matter further to clarify key points.

Whether you're in discussion with your family members, friends, coworkers, or the person you hope will soon hire you, the art of communicating effectively will always serve you well.

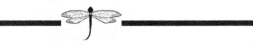

Takeaway:

Communicating effectively strengthens relationships!

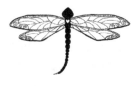

Rule 6:

Appreciate the Human Touch

You may remember when you'd glide your car into a gas station and switch the key off. The attendants would fill your tank, check under the hood, wash your windshields, and sweep the interior. When you drove off, your car was cared for, and you basked in the attentive service.

If you didn't experience these personalized services, you may be more accustomed to today's near-complete automation. Our world is full of touch screens, sensory-activated devices, and camera-driven technology. And there's an app for virtually everything!

Technology rules the day and can sometimes seem to control us. We have "buds" in our ears, smart watches that prompt our activities, GPS devices that give us directions, and cell phones, laptops, or iPads that know more than we can comprehend in a lifetime.

While we appreciate conveniences such as self-roaming vacuum cleaners, we may notice that advancing technology has fostered a certain dehumanization as well. While automation streamlines many services, there is nothing better than knowing someone cares about your unique needs.

Consider how you interact with others. Do you choose emails and texts over a phone call or in-person meeting? Have you been in the same building with a friend and used texting or instant messaging to communicate? Do you patronize stores that provide exceptional, personalized service for important purchases?

The human touch is warmer, friendlier, and often more helpful than an electronic bleep. Recognize the value that full service offers and seek out ways to provide the human touch in your interactions with others whenever possible.

Takeaway:

Add a personal touch!

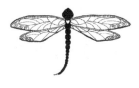

Rule 7:

Ensure Quality Time

We all know that quality time is important. But if you bring it up in conversation, you'll soon find that people have different ideas about what this concept entails and how it works. For example, is it quality time if you and your family are watching a movie together, and it's so riveting that you don't talk throughout it? What if you make time for friends by inviting them to an event that you really want to attend (though it is less desirable for the friends)? What if you're sharing a meal with another but are periodically checking your cell phone?

According to one dictionary, *quality time* is "time spent giving all of one's attention to someone who is close." In another dictionary, the focus is on the goal: "time that you spend with someone doing enjoyable things together so that your relationship remains strong."

In order to share quality time with someone, you'll want to focus on mutually enjoyable activities and eliminate cell phone use and other distractions. In conversation, remember that the very best gift you can give someone is the purity of your attention. Proactively focusing on the conversation and the body language of the person you are communicating with is critical to connecting and bonding.

Consider suggesting an activity that is more important to the other person than to yourself and develop an appreciation for what they most enjoy. Then, be present by making eye contact, paying attention, and staying in the moment to promote healthy and welcoming relationships that enhance your life.

Takeaway:

Focus on the relationship that's right in front of you!

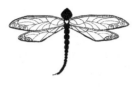

Rule 8:

Give Back

So often these days we hear the terms *giving back* and *paying it forward*. A football player donates millions to a children's hospital. Huge corporate gifts go to Africa for building homes and schools. Charitable enterprises pop up like flowers to sponsor projects and to support others when natural disasters strike. These good-will gestures are as needed as they are wonderful!

As individuals, we may feel that we don't have meaningful impact on large-scale situations. But what each of us *can* do is to *share* what we do have. Remember that taken together, our small donations do indeed significantly support our community's needs.

The foundation to giving back is based on the *Golden Rule*. The *Golden Rule* has stood the test of time and still remains the essence of doing good for others. We feel a warm satisfaction from knowing that our gifts contribute to improving the lives of others.

Opportunities to give back or pay it forward range from simple gestures, such as holding the door for the person behind us or speaking kindly to someone in distress to more time-consuming activities such as donating clothes and household items to charity and volunteering at a local foodbank or animal shelter.

There will always be so many ways we can give back or pay it forward. When we do, we become part of a much larger and united effort to change the world. Then, we can share in the hope that tomorrow will be a better day.

So, offer what you can to help others, both monetarily and by your actions—and savor the joy that comes from following the *Golden Rule*.

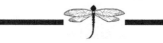

Takeaway:

Do unto others!

Part Four:

Rules for Enjoying Healthy Living

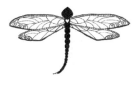

Rule 1:

Exercise Regularly

Great news! Regular daily exercise is extremely beneficial for enjoying a long, healthy life! It has been shown that calorie-burning exercise can reduce obesity, heart disease, and its relatives—stroke, high blood pressure, and high cholesterol, as well as the incidence of diabetes, depression, and dementia.

To contribute to your good health, exercise on a regular basis as opposed to occasionally. There's no single form of exercise that's appropriate for everyone. You have complete control over what exercises you do, so be sure to select the form(s) that you enjoy the most. Whether it's walking, swimming, biking, golfing, playing tennis, strength training, rowing, kayaking, rock climbing, yoga, Pilates, etc., pick your favorites—variety is the spice of life! Whether you exercise alone or with others, enjoy activities as part of your daily routine.

Regular exercise isn't about trying to look like you could pose on stage in a Speedo or a bikini; it's about developing your muscles and strength. There are practical and proven health advantages to increasing your lean muscle tissue, including decreasing your body fat and giving you a leaner appearance. New lean muscle may also actually help to improve your balance and may lessen the likelihood of falls, as well as improve your heart health. Increased strength and conditioning may also prevent exercise-induced injuries.

The benefits that you will obtain from exercising will be supplemented by the joy that comes with staying active and doing things that bring you pleasure. So, exercise regularly to reap the many health benefits and enjoy your favorite activities each day.

Takeaway:

Let's get moving!

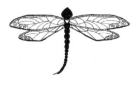

Rule 2:

Eat Smart

G ood news! Smart eating doesn't imply crash dieting. In fact, as most fitness gurus will attest, diets don't often work to improve your overall health. Anyone who has yo-yo dieted can confirm that statement. Why? First off, diets can reduce your muscle mass, which lowers your metabolism. Second, diets may reduce your bone density and water, which are essential to your health. Third, the weight you lose while dieting is often regained—as body fat.

If you want to lose body fat and keep it off, it must be replaced simultaneously with new lean muscle tissue. To do this, you have to work it off!

There are many reasons why people may become out of shape. Whether you may have a medical condition, physical limitations, or little time for healthy food preparation or exercise, it can be challenging to stay fit. It takes self-discipline to learn new ways of eating and develop exercise habits needed to stay healthy.

Both *what you eat* and *how much you eat* determines your current weight as well as your ability to maintain your long-term health. Nutrition experts recommend consuming a variety of fresh fruits, vegetables and nuts; a variety of whole grain breads, cereals, and rice; skim, 1 percent, or soy milk; olive and canola oils; and plenty of water. They also stipulate that you should avoid or limit simple carbohydrates (crackers, cookies, chips, pastries, etc.); sodas and sugar; whole or 2 percent milk; meat (beef, pork, bacon, ham, etc.); salt; and alcoholic beverages (to no more than one or two drinks per day).

So, eat smarter to improve your health.

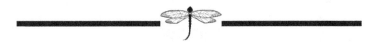

Takeaway:

Bon appetite!
Cheers to your health!

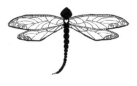

Rule 3:

Get Enough Sleep

D o you struggle with getting a good night's sleep? If so, you've likely heard advice such as "maintain a consistent schedule, establish a pre-bed routine, refrain from eating and drinking the hour or two before tucking yourself in, ensure the bedroom is cool and dark, etc." While these rules are good suggestions, they may not always ensure restful slumber.

Some of us seem to be genetically predisposed to needing only five to seven hours of sleep to be physically and cognitively alert. Others require a solid eight hours of sleep to be able to function at peak performance. Regardless of the number of hours we sleep, experiencing deep, restful sleep is essential to fully enjoying each day.

Given the many daily responsibilities you have, you may struggle to fall asleep because your mind is racing at bedtime. Try to calm yourself by adopting relaxation techniques, such as diaphragmatic breathing or progressive relaxation, to help you drift comfortably off to sleep. Praying and counting your blessings may also help to clear your mind to fall asleep peacefully.

If you tend to fall asleep readily but wake up in the middle of the night with something important on your mind, consider writing it down. This allows your mind to rest, knowing it won't be forgotten the next morning.

Take time to identify what calms and relaxes you the most and add that to your nightly routine. Many people discover that use of sleep sound machines enable more restorative sleep. If deep sleep eludes you for too long, consider taking a power nap now and then until you are back on track.

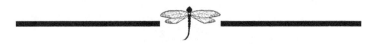

Takeaway:

Goodnight, sweet dreams!

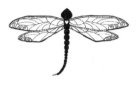

Rule 4:

Stay Active

We live in a predominantly sedentary culture. We sit while eating, driving, working, and watching TV shows or sports. We often sit in a bent-forward position that can be detrimental over time. Maintaining proper alignment and strong back muscles is critical for many exercises. Practicing good posture and exercising regularly can help you to maintain fitness throughout your life.

As with any regular activity, it takes motivation and discipline to stay fit. Watch TV while lying on the couch, or go for a thirty-minute walk? It's entirely up to you! It is commonly understood that walking, with good posture and a clear mind, can improve many health conditions, such as weight management, high blood pressure, heart disease, bone density, coordination, mood disorders, and more. So, choose to engage, stand as tall as you can, and get moving!

In order to stay active, consider making it part of your daily routine. Identify several physical activities that you enjoy the most, then commit to engaging in them on a weekly basis. When you truly enjoy an activity, you are much more likely to build it into your routine. By rotating among these activities, you will decrease the likelihood of becoming bored and making excuses to avoid exercise. Many people also find that exercising with others helps them to stay committed as well.

Once you include physical activities in your schedule, they'll require no more planning or thought than any of your other daily habits. You'll reach a level of consistency with exercise that will help you to maintain an active lifestyle—and you'll look positively at this decision!

Takeaway:

Enjoy activities that get you moving!

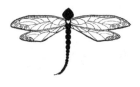

Rule 5:

Maintain a Balanced Lifestyle

Have you ever felt as if one aspect of your life is consuming all of your time or energy? This imbalanced feeling is uncomfortable and happens to all of us periodically, on a situational basis. However, if this continues too long, you may feel that your quality of life has diminished.

Sometimes, challenging situations build up gradually and go unnoticed until we feel overwhelmed. To avoid this, periodically ask yourself how happy you are in your current situation. Consider how well your needs are being met in each of the following areas: physical, mental, spiritual, emotional, social, environmental, and financial well-being. Perhaps seek input from the key people in your life (family, friends, managers, coworkers, neighbors, etc.) to help you to prioritize your efforts and identify potential changes you may want to make.

To achieve a healthy balance, be sure to factor in the amount of time you'd like for your own personal interests, while preserving some "downtime" to rest and refresh your spirit. If feeling overwhelmed, eliminate those activities that are of lowest priority to you and to others. And be sure that you don't take on more responsibilities than you know you can successfully handle. After all, stress management techniques are wonderful, but they aren't miracle workers and can't provide balance in your lifestyle.

So, listen to your feelings, identify the source of undue stress in any one area, and make changes as needed to improve the quality of your daily life. With a healthy, well-balanced lifestyle, you'll be better able to cope with challenges and experience more peace and satisfaction in your life.

Takeaway:

Everything in moderation!

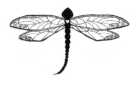

Rule 6:

Embrace Your Changing Body

Have you ever wondered what "aging gracefully" means? Aging gracefully entails accepting your changing body while being able to continue enjoying the activities that please you the most. It also includes being at peace with any unavoidable limitations you may have or develop as you age. A primary goal as we age is to maintain a healthy lifestyle, which includes eating a well-balanced, nutritious diet, receiving all recommended preventative healthcare, and proactively managing health concerns as soon as they arise.

So much of what we negatively call "aging" is simply the reduction in the intensity level of our physical activity. However, you can address this by switching to lower-impact forms of activities. While *some* of your health conditions may be due to genetics, you have substantial influence over whether your later years are spent enjoying life or are spent with pain, discomfort, and possible dependence on others.

Some people are acutely aware of the unavoidable impact that aging has on their appearance. You can dye your hair or have a facelift or a tummy tuck to *appear* younger, typically without any impact on your overall health. While looking better may boost your confidence level, there are far more important issues at hand, such as feeling better, moving comfortably, maintaining your energy level, and living pain-free to best enjoy the twilight of your life.

There's also the day-to-day joy of not just feeling good physically but continuing to be an active family member, employee, or citizen. There is no better path to high self-esteem than knowing that you're responsibly caring for your health and continuing to enjoy your life.

Takeaway:

Appreciate and take care of yourself!

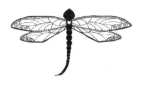

Rule 7:

Develop a Positive Outlook

Have you ever stopped to consider your outlook on life? Most of us desire a positive attitude toward life, a "glass half-full" approach toward ourselves and others. In order to achieve this, we must accept our limitations and realize that disappointment is a natural part of life. We need to come to terms with the fact that life is not always fair. How you react during challenging moments reveals your character. Having a positive outlook helps you to move beyond your setbacks and live a happier, more peaceful life.

A positive self-image is essential to having a good outlook on life. Enhance your self-esteem by reflecting regularly on your strengths and talents and recognizing how you've grown through past mistakes. In relationships with others, offer your unique gifts and accept theirs. Nurture healthy relationships that enhance your self-esteem and bring out the best in you.

Maintaining a positive attitude is easier to do when considering your own unique self as opposed to comparing your situation with the lives of others. Think about the struggles you face that are invisible to the outside world, and know that others have invisible issues of their own to deal with. Having a positive attitude enables us to choose to be happy in life. A positive outlook helps us to live each day to the fullest! While it is good to remember lessons learned from the past and to maintain hope for the future, be sure to live in the moment and recognize it as the precious gift it truly is.

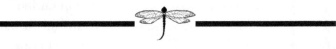

Takeaway:

Keep your glass half-full!

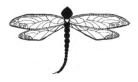

Rule 8:

Take Care of Yourself

You can try so hard to be healthy. You can choose to eat the most nutritious foods and avoid consuming alcohol and cigarettes. You may spend forty-five minutes a day exercising to improve your cardiovascular system. You can even work diligently on building muscle strength with three workouts a week. And you may try to avoid stress and get plenty of restful sleep.

Diligent though we are, the aging process affects us all. As you age, your hair may fall out or lose its color, your teeth and gums may show degeneration, your eyesight may change, your hearing may lessen, and genetic inheritance may cause your heart or another organ's function to be suboptimal. While some of these health conditions are considered *normal* as you get older, you need to take care of yourself to enjoy life as fully as possible at every age.

In addition to doing what you can on your own, preventive medical care is needed to ensure that you remain healthy. This includes having annual physicals, routine dental, vision, and hearing exams, receiving pertinent vaccines, and getting mammograms and colonoscopies as indicated. Prevention is one of the best ways to take good care of your health.

Along the way, accidents may happen. You may break an ankle while stepping off the curb onto those quaint cobblestones while visiting Charleston, or experience back pain while picking up your well-fed grandchild. Take all accidents seriously, as they may cause impacts to your body that are invisible to the untrained eye. Life happens, and you must take care of yourself and roll with the punches.

Takeaway:

Look out for number one!

Part Five:

Rules for Enjoying the Seasons

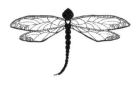

Rule 1:

Make Resolutions

As each new year begins, do you reflect on the past and project into the future? Do you contemplate what you learned from the previous year? Do you think about what the coming year has in store for you and what you really want out of life? These considerations are essential for making New Year's resolutions.

January is the perfect time to think about what we might want to change in our lives and commit to a resolution. If you've attempted resolutions in the past and failed to keep them, consider simplifying or right-sizing your goal to make this year's more attainable. Ensure that the goal is personally important and commit to it from the heart. Then set up ways to measure your success along the journey to achieving the goal. Be sure to celebrate your progress along the way!

Perhaps you want to share your feelings and deepen your connections with family or friends, explore new and beautiful places together, improve your communication skills, or spend more time in reflection. Regardless of the goal, be thankful that each new day you can assess your progress and modify your actions if needed to better achieve that goal. Search your heart for a resolution concerning an important relationship in your life, perhaps with your own personal habits, with God or with others. As that relationship improves, you'll likely feel more peace and contentment than you did before.

So, take the time and make the effort to improve a significant relationship and enhance your enjoyment of a beautiful new year!

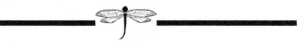

Takeaway:

Make this year the best!

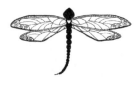

Rule 2:

Treasure Valentine's Day

I n February, we pay homage to St. Valentine, the patron
saint of romantic and courtly love. With cards, choc-
olate, flowers, candlelight dinners, and sparkly gifts,
we celebrate with our sweethearts on this day set aside for
l'amour. Love is the diamond of emotions because it is so
multifaceted and priceless!

In our everyday lives, we use the word *love* frequently,
as in "I'd love another piece of candy" or "Love ya," which
has become a popular farewell. And what about songs?
There are so many songs in existence that include love as
a theme.

Let's reflect on how that sweet emotion of love per-
meates all areas of our lives. We love our family members
and may consider them our mainstays in life. We love our
friends as they add color to our lives. We love our pets, and
we grow in love through leisure time and favorite activities
that nourish our bodies, minds, and spirits.

We extend our love as we care for the homeless, the
hungry, the ill, and those whose lives become ravaged by
war or natural disasters.

So, make Valentine's Day bigger than romance. Appreciate the bounty of love you have in your life. Recognize that love is the ultimate gift and every day you can give and receive it freely.

Be sure to share your gift of love with kind words and attentive listening to your family, friends, work associates, and everyone you meet. Your example will encourage others to do the same!

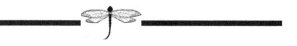

Takeaway:

Spread love!

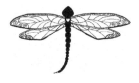

Rule 3:

Embrace Spring Fever

Depending on where you live, March or April teases us with token warm, sunny days which suggest that spring is here. Finally, we open our windows and enjoy fresh air sweeping through our homes or search the garden for the first crocus or the tips of daffodils popping through the dried leaves. We feel energized and happily return to outdoor walks and sports activities. Many of us may feel the urge to clean our homes, including even a closet or two.

Spring has become the season for clean-up—the time to sort through closets that may be virtual time capsules. Fashions can quickly go out of style . . . but often return decades later. So, consider keeping a select few of the fashion items you absolutely adore.

And then there's the closet with photo albums, boxes of pictures destined for digitizing, and various mementos. Isn't it easy to get caught in "a quick look" that lasts the entire afternoon?

Spring is the time to air out our most fervent desires as well as our homes. After the hibernation of winter, we are ready to refresh our routines. It's the perfect time to plan picnics, vacations, staycations, and celebrations with family and friends.

Springtime is when we feel a special anticipation of the months to come, as the world blossoms forth with infinite magic. Our souls are nourished, and we feel energized to fulfill our hopes and dreams in a new way. This mood enhancement is often called spring fever, as it can spread easily to those around us. So, breathe deeply, share freely, and enjoy renewed energy for life!

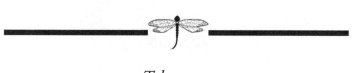

Takeaway:

Spring into action!

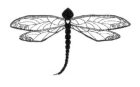

Rule 4:

Appreciate Your Mother and Father

To honor your mother and father, reflect on what their legacy has been for you, what you appreciate the most, and how their guiding light has enriched your life. You may remember them laughing, playing music, serving others, and simply enjoying life. Hopefully, these memories fill you with a surge of warmth and love.

Were you raised according to the *Golden Rule*—to treat people just the way you want to be treated, with respect, compassion, and sincerity? Hopefully, your parents instilled in you a sense of responsibility and the desire to put your best effort into everything you do. Perhaps your parents promoted accomplishment, not only in school but also in life—and taught you that continuous learning and sharing with others are gifts you actually give to yourself.

Hopefully, your parents encouraged you to have confidence in yourself to enable you to reach any goal and accomplish your dreams. And most likely, your parents took pride in watching you grow and become ever more aware and appreciative of the role you play in the beautiful world we live in.

Parents want to pass on the important qualities that help us reach our full potential and wrap them up like little gifts to be passed on to our own children and others around us. This is how we all can leave a legacy and positively impact the world around us.

So, honor your parents with all your heart for their love and faith in you. And beam with pride when you see the strong values you've been taught displayed by your children.

Takeaway:

Pass on your legacy!

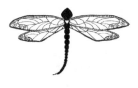

Rule 5:

Savor Summertime

What's another word for summer? *Fun!* It's a time to turn our backs to the indoors and step outside to feel the warmth and glow that beautiful summer days present to us each year. It's the time to enjoy the sound of ice cubes in lemonade, tea, or margaritas and the aroma of fresh-cut grass or our favorite foods cooking on the grill. Summer also provides us with the unleashed beauty of the great outdoors with trees in full leaf, gardens bursting with color, and dramatic sunsets of glorious beauty.

For many of us, summer is equated with more family time. Whether family traditions include vacations, trips to the beach, or having regular picnics, many of us enjoy getting the entire clan together. During summer, children especially enjoy time to rest, play, and relax in their favorite ways. For many, the less-structured time is refreshing and promotes learning and growing through different activities and interactions.

Summer offers outdoor concerts, lawn parties, celebrations of weddings and family reunions, visits from cherished friends, or just long walks with those we love. These are the activities we yearned for on cold winter nights. Summer also provides time to read a good book from a hammock, porch swing, or beach blanket, and to rest, listening to the sound of the songbirds or watching the sun set over the water. Summer's sensual, restful pleasures reveal themselves best when the sky is bright and the air is balmy.

Summer is when Mother Nature takes us by the hand and offers us the joy of communing with her through countless outdoor experiences and adventures.

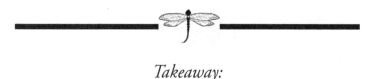

Takeaway:

Enjoy sunshine and fun time!

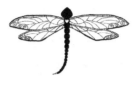

Rule 6:

Appreciate Autumn

Where summer found many of you vacationing far from home, fall is a time to appreciate the joys available in your own backyard. Depending on where you live, autumn produces such splendor as the trees transition from green to a variety of warm, golden hues of yellow, orange, red, and brown. This scenic transition eventually produces a floor of fallen crispy brown leaves that crunch underfoot. The fallen leaves are perfect for kids of all ages to scoop up and toss into the air, creating a marvelous overhead shower or to gather into piles that are perfect for jumping in.

As you appreciate the beauty of God's paintbrush of autumn colors, you may also enjoy warm, sunny days with crisp, cool nights. Fall beckons us to enjoy a variety of outdoor activities, such as fall festivals, oyster roasts, football games, tailgate parties, planting spring bulbs in the garden, or hiking on a nature trail.

Autumn is a magical time to celebrate harvest by visiting a pumpkin farm or cider mill or enjoying a hayride. It's a time to spend with family and friends, either inside near a warm fireplace or at an outside bonfire or firepit. It's the time for sipping hot drinks such as hot spiced cider and pumpkin spiced lattes—or cool white wines from a recent grape harvest.

Halloween fun brings spooky haunted houses, costume parties, and delightful trick-or-treating. And, of course, it's the season to munch on candy corn, caramel apples, donuts, and bite-sized Halloween candy. Enjoy!

So, keep your eyes open wide and appreciate the glorious scenery and joys a plentiful harvest brings each year.

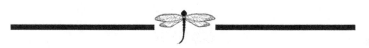

Takeaway:

Enjoy an abundant harvest!

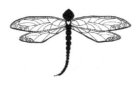

Rule 7:

Give Thanks

Thanksgiving is the uniquely American holiday that touches on the values most people cherish— being with family, reflecting on our blessings, and expressing our gratitude for the bounty bestowed upon us. But beyond the family gatherings and the bountiful table, there's much we can be thankful for. We can be grateful for each day of life on earth, for the miracle of creation that surrounds us, and for our family, friends, neighbors, and coworkers.

Across the land, Thanksgiving is a day of expressing thanks by serving. Volunteers all over America join forces with Foodbanks, Meals on Wheels, area restaurants, and service organizations to magically transform church social halls and neighborhood gathering places into dining rooms, cafeterias, and banquet facilities. Here they will serve opulent feasts for the hungry, the needy, the homeless, and those who are alone.

These special volunteers may spend their day slicing turkey, manning the gravy ladle, scooping dressing, spooning sweet potatoes, or doling out cranberry sauce to bring Thanksgiving to neighbors for whom this would be just another day of hardship or uncertainty.

Thanksgiving is a wonderful time for togetherness and for bonding with those you love. While we've been blessed, we sense the inequalities of life and recognize our responsibility to help with improvements. So, be a friend and a volunteer to make things better. Be the one who listens and lends a hand to create laughter to shine a light in the lives of others. And always be thankful you can do it.

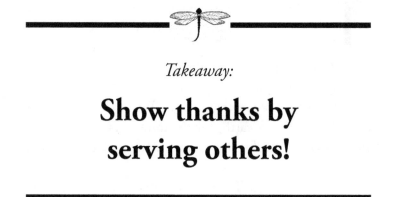

Takeaway:

Show thanks by serving others!

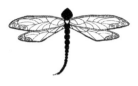

Rule 8:

Enjoy the Holidays

Every holiday season, most of us ramp up our shopping! Over the years, have you taxed your imagination for just the right gifts that will bring a sparkle to the eyes of each recipient? And each holiday season, does it get more difficult? How can we make gift-giving simpler and more meaningful?

You become the holiday gift! Giving the gift of oneself only requires a little forethought, a little time, and a lot of love. This ensures your gift is personalized, useful, and something your recipient will remember. It's from the heart and unlikely to be duplicated by others.

You may offer to babysit for a young mother so she can enjoy a free afternoon, prepare a meal for busy friends, care for pets, mow the lawn for neighbors who are away, or shop for an elderly family member or friend.

Perhaps you have special keepsakes that you would like to share with a friend or loved one. A special piece of jewelry, a money clip, or a belt buckle can become a token of love that will touch one's heart and become a legacy gift.

Spend time thinking about the true meaning of gift-giving. Gifts do not always have to be objects or edibles. When you provide a personal service, your gift reflects your love and concern for another. These gifts can bring joy, leave a longer lasting impression, and inspire others to give of themselves as well. Give holiday gifts to fill the hearts of both the giver and receiver with joy, gifts that keep on giving.

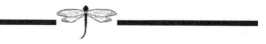

Takeaway:

The best gift is yourself!

Rule Notes

Rule Notes

About the Authors

Sylvia Weinstein Craft is publisher and editor of *Oyster Pointer*, an award-winning feature newspaper and primary source of "good news" information for the city of Newport News, Virginia. Prior to launching *Oyster Pointer* in 1986, Sylvia spent twenty-six years with the Virginia Peninsula Industrial Council (VPIC), an organization devoted to improving the community through economic development, where she was the council's director of public relations for eleven years.

A true entrepreneur, Sylvia formed her own public relations, advertising, and marketing agency, which later became The Weinstein Agency, a successful business garnering many international and national awards.

Sylvia attended The College of William & Mary and has been serving her community as an exemplary role model for decades, receiving numerous awards including a Humanitarian Award presented by the Virginia Center for Inclusive Communities, for her community involvement, professional leadership, and lifetime of contributions to improving the lives of others.

Sylvia resides in Newport News, Virginia.

Dr. Lisa Spiller is Distinguished Professor of Marketing, Emerita in the Joseph W. Luter, III School of Business at Christopher Newport University (CNU) in Newport News, Virginia. An inspiring teacher, mentor, advisor, and role model to her students and junior faculty, Dr. Spiller had a profound impact on the lives of many during her thirty-one-year career at CNU prior to her retirement in 2022.

Dr. Spiller has garnered more than forty honors and awards for her extraordinary achievement, leadership, and valuable contributions to her students, university, discipline, and community. An accomplished scholar, Dr. Spiller authored several college textbooks, including *Selling and Sales Management: Developing Skills for Success* and *Direct, Digital & Data-Driven Marketing,* both published by SAGE.

Prior to joining the CNU faculty, Lisa was a faculty member at Avila College in Missouri and the University of Missouri-Kansas City. She also served as marketing director with a McDonald's Restaurant franchise in Erie, Pennsylvania, prior to her career in academia. Spiller received her BS in business administration and her MBA from Gannon University in Erie, Pennsylvania, and her PhD from the University of Missouri-Kansas City.

Lisa resides in Newport News, Virginia.

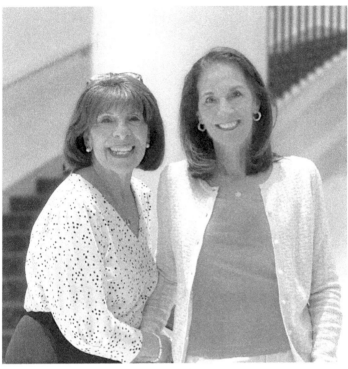

Sylvia and Lisa

A free ebook edition is available with the purchase of this book.

To claim your free ebook edition:

1. Visit MorganJamesBOGO.com
2. Sign your name CLEARLY in the space
3. Complete the form and submit a photo of the entire copyright page
4. You or your friend can download the ebook to your preferred device

Morgan James
BOGO™

A **FREE** ebook edition is available for you or a friend with the purchase of this print book.

CLEARLY SIGN YOUR NAME ABOVE

Instructions to claim your free ebook edition:
1. Visit MorganJamesBOGO.com
2. Sign your name CLEARLY in the space above
3. Complete the form and submit a photo of this entire page
4. You or your friend can download the ebook to your preferred device

Print & Digital Together Forever.

Snap a photo   Free ebook   Read anywhere

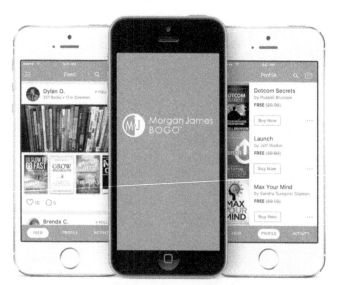

Printed in the USA
CPSIA information can be obtained
at www.ICGtesting.com
JSHW021510150923
48595JS00002B/24

9 781636 982144